# INTIMACY II
## WITHOUT RESPONSIBILITY
The Conscious Evolution of Love

**Wendyne Limber**, MA, LMFT, RDT-BCT

Copyright ©2010 by
Wendyne McGowen Limber

Cover Art: Samantha Nagel
Book Design: Aaron Welch, bigA Designs & Printing

All rights reserved. No part of this publication may be reproduced or transmitted in any form or by any means, electronic or mechanical, including photocopy, without permission in writing from Wendyne Limber. However, if you really love this book and you want to copy one of these pages, then please do and pass it forward.

ISBN: 978-0-557-73691-1

Printed in the United States of America

**Dedicated to**
*Lesley, Elijah, Hilary and Vanessa*

# Table of Contents

| | | |
|---|---|---|
| **Introduction** | I Was Just Thinking | 6 |
| **Chapter One** | I Am Speaking My Truth | 9 |
| **Chapter Two** | Embracing Feelings | 25 |
| **Chapter Three** | Wound Re-Enactment | 41 |
| **Chapter Four** | Intimacy Boundaries | 57 |
| **Chapter Five** | Responsibility vs. Blame | 73 |
| **Chapter Six** | Letting Love In | 89 |
| **Chapter Seven** | The Evolution of Love | 105 |
| **Epilogue • AND** | | 121 |
| **About the Author** | | 124 |
| **Acknowledgements** | | 128 |

I was just thinking...

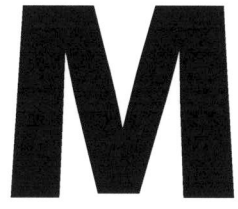aybe I'll write a book tonight, because I have the freedom and the passion to do so. Maybe tonight will be the night that all the words come easily and effortlessly... I shall know and hear and write whatever the universe is wanting me to know.

Maybe I'll write a book tonight, because tonight I have given myself the gift of alone time and I feel the passion of the words in my fingers and heart. I have been waiting for this day for a long time, not knowing that tonight, might be the night that it would happen.

Maybe I'll write a book tonight that could be the culmination of what I have been learning all these years... all about being free and loving myself and giving myself permission to be real and open and intimate and responsible to *me*. Yes, I love the idea of really taking care of myself instead of taking care of everyone or anyone else.

Maybe I'll write a book tonight—a book that would help people heal and transform their ideas about love and intimacy and relationship. I have always loved deeply. That has been my strength and my weakness, for many times, I have given up my own Self to help save someone else.

And somewhere I forgot that we all are on our own path and it is not my job to save someone else. And today I know, that when I was saving someone else, I accidentally thought it was me.

Maybe tonight....

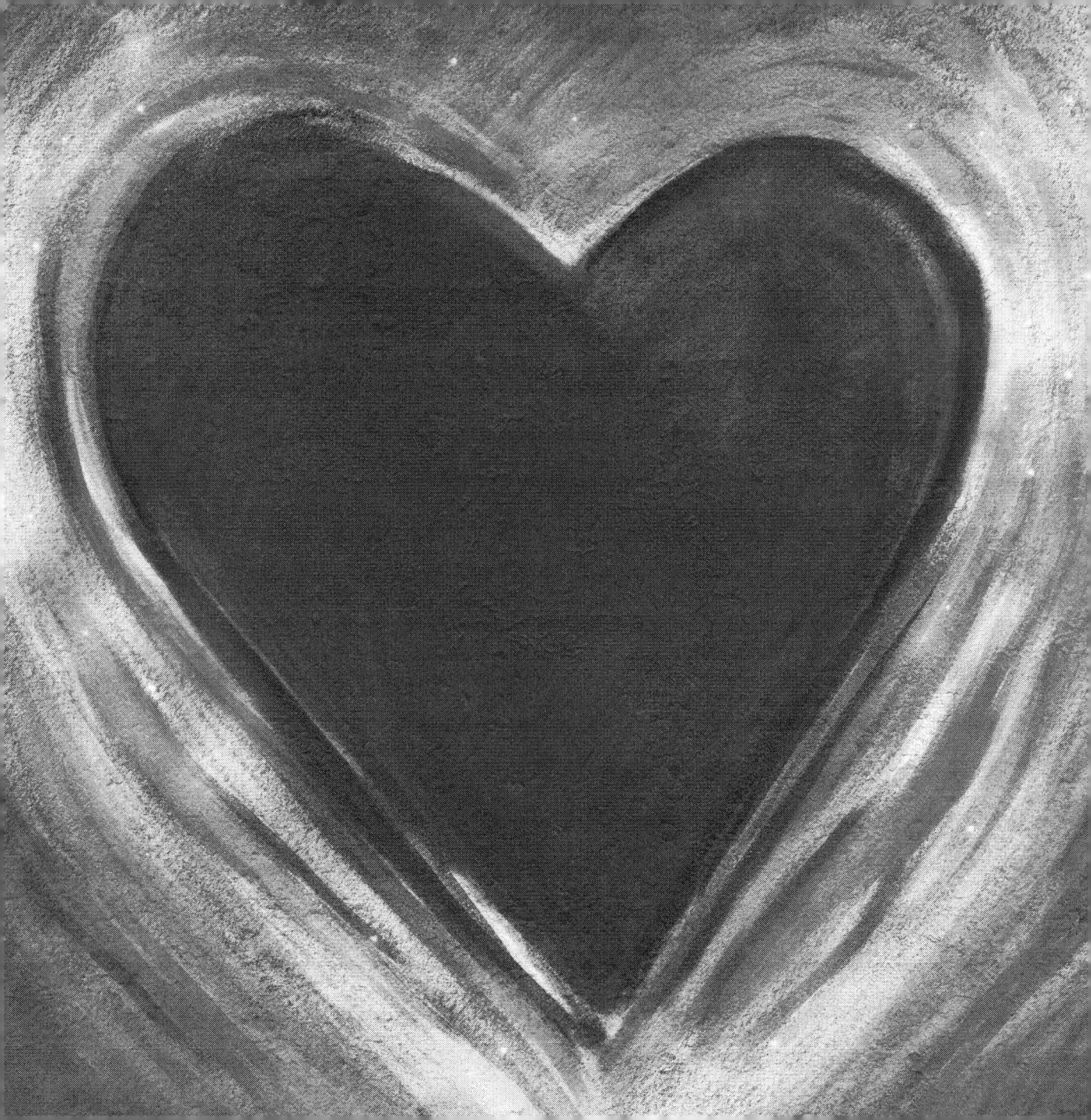

# CHAPTER ONE

I Am Speaking My Truth

# Principle #1

I am here on this earth for my own soul's evolution...
I am not here to take care of *you*.

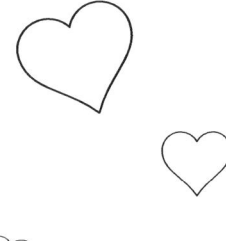

Love is not about taking care of someone else. Even though taking care of someone else could be rewarding, it usually becomes a burden sooner or later. Some people learned to do this, because they had to, in order to survive. Some children grew up too fast—having to take care of their siblings or emotionally unbalanced parents.

Care-taking can become a disease. Most caretakers become martyrs and eventually become sick or addicted to something to take away the pain. When I care-take someone else, I get to *not take care* of myself. If I am care-taking, *you* are what I am always thinking about. I begin to worry, control, manipulate and hold in my feelings, *or* I become angry and hurtful. Either way, it does not work, and I am not whole.

*I am here on this earth for my own soul's evolution. I am here to take care of ME. And, I will let YOU take care of yourself. This does not mean that I will not help you or support you. I will figure out HOW to do that in the healthiest way that serves us both.*

*As I learn to TAKE CARE OF ME, I am actually more free to love you fully. I will not have to be fearful of the time we spend together, knowing that I am not giving away a part of myself. Today I commit to my own journey.*

## Principle #2

When I take responsibility for your feelings or your happiness, I am taking away a piece of you, leaving you helpless.

**responsibility** • noun (pl. -ties) *(Wikipedia)*
the state or fact of having a duty to deal with something or of having control over someone: women bear children and take responsibility for child care.

- the state or fact of being accountable or to blame for something: the group has claimed responsibility for a string of murders.
- the opportunity or ability to act independently and make decisions without authorization: we would expect individuals lower down the organization to take on more responsibility.
- (often responsibilities) a thing that one is required to do as part of a job, role, or legal obligation: he will take over the responsibilities of overseas director.
- [in sing.] (responsibility to/toward) a moral obligation to behave correctly toward or in respect of: individuals have a responsibility to control personal behavior.

*I would never want to take responsibility for your feelings. My goodness, it would take away your very core human self. If I did all that according to definition, you would never learn to be in your own power. I would leave you helpless, and you would have learned it from me!*

*And surely, I do not want control over you, or moral obligation or being accountable or blamed if everything does not work out according to MY plan for you. I am RESPONSIBLE for my own healthy body, mind, and spirit. Today I am willing to let go of taking responsibility for your happiness and your life. I am doing all I can to let go and allow whatever is to happen to happen.*

## Principle #3

I can love you and really tell you my truth
without being *responsible* for your reaction.

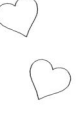

The greatest freedom in the world is being able to be emotionally honest with others and myself. When I can express my real feelings, my body is so happy and healthy. If I hold in my real feelings because I am afraid of your reaction, I am not being real or honest or authentic, and I begin to lose parts of myself.

When I begin to hold in and hold on, I live in my secret self. Sometimes your pain is so scary to me that I just do not want to say something that will create pain for you because I am afraid of your reaction. I do not like to see you sad. I do not like to feel your anger because that really scares me.

At some time in my life I got the impression I had the power to make you happy or sad, and that even extended to my believing at times that I could be responsible for your life or death. Way too much for me! I now see my belief was in error. I forgive whoever helped me take that on.

*I want to experience real love with you, which means that I will tell you my true feelings, my truth—without fear of your reaction. If you do have a reaction, I will know that it is ABOUT YOU. And, that YOU must be responsible for your own feelings and reactions. I can only be me.*

*I give myself permission today to speak my truth in ways I have not done before. I let go of my secrets and will work with my own pain, as I realize it is really my own pain that I am afraid of, not yours. I let go of taking responsibility for how you may react to my truth, even if this is scary and painful for me.*

## Principle #4

When I try to shield you from pain or hurt feelings,
I am really taking away your power or
taking away your opportunity to discover your power.

It is perfectly healthy to *care* about how someone feels. Most humans genuinely care about other people's pain and sorrow. And we all want to be happy and wish for our loved ones to be happy.

The thing is, we are all here on our own journey through life, in order to evolve our soul. Opportunities arise all the time for people to discover their deeper powers. Pain, challenge, change, sorrow, loss and grief are often the thing that opens a person to their inner power and strength. When I shield my loved one from pain or hurt, I am taking away their opportunity to discover their greatness!

*Therefore, I am committed to NOT shielding you from the natural consequences of your actions, or from the painful events and happenings in your life. I commit to facing my own pain and working with it, and letting you do the same.*

*Somehow it seems that when I let go and let you feel and be in your pain fully, you are the one who learns how to solve your problems, discover your inner and outer resources, fix things and advance through your life. If I save or shield you from the repercussion of your actions, you never fully birth yourself, and you may feel the power of moving through your dark night of the soul.*

*I want you to know that I will be here if you need me to hold you while you are crying your sacred tears, but I may not hand you a Kleenex, unless you ask. I commit to practicing this way of thinking, being and doing, so that I can really follow through with this most important principle when the time comes. And, it will.*

## Principle #5

The more I believe that you are a certain way, the more I prove it to myself. I gather evidence always to prove my belief.

Whatever I believe about you, I will prove. If I believe that you do not love me, then I will gather evidence to prove that. If I believe that you are abandoning me, then I will surely find the facts to prove it! If I believe you are hurting me, then I will show you a list of all the times that happened.

My perception of everything—how I view you and my world, is based on what I believe. My perceptions become my truth, because that is my only experience. Your perceptions are your truth because that is your only experience. And, whatever it is you keep in your mind, eventually will come to pass. And then we will gather evidence to *prove it.*

In loving relationships, it is common for one person to feel abandoned and "needy"—really craving nurturing, attention and love. Not by accident, the other person may tend to feel enmeshed and smothered, wanting and needing more space. This is a classic relationship pattern. Two people often come together and fit into this pattern like a puzzle!

*For me to experience* Intimacy without Responsibility, *I must become conscious of my core beliefs and be willing to understand how I project those beliefs on others, especially those I am close to.*

*When I am willing to look inside at my core beliefs, issues and needs, I will understand my perceptions and need to prove what I believe about you! If you do the same, we will really understand each other's perceptions, and that will make it easier to really communicate and move toward emotional intimacy.*

## Principle #6

It is my wish and desire that you will not spare me your truth, either. It is more important to me that you speak your truth and your real feelings, rather than trying to protect me from pain or hurt.

All of this sounds very freeing and exciting, right? And guess what... it applies to *me* too!

*Intimacy without Responsibility* also means that I am willing to hear your truth about me. I am willing to take responsibility for my own feelings. You are not hurting me, rather I am choosing to be hurt by certain words or actions or ways of being.

If I blame you for the way I feel, I am giving away my power. If I need you to be a certain way or do a certain thing to make me feel better, I am not taking the responsibility for my own journey.

*So, please do not spare me your truth. Tell me how you feel and be honest with me about your life. I am healing and transforming myself every day, and even if I do feel hurt, I will be okay. Being hurt or hearing your truth may be the best thing that ever happened to me.*

*Please allow me to be powerful and vulnerable at the same time. Believe that I will not die or kill myself because you are not feeling or doing something that I wish you would. You are not in charge of my life or death.*

*I am learning the art and skill of speaking my truth and I want the opportunity to grow and be with an authentic person who also speaks their truth. Please be completely honest with me. I can feel it inside when you are not, anyway. And so can you. I commit today to risk being real.*

## Principle #7

I am making a choice to take care of myself now...
to really be true to my own passions and inner guidance.
When I am true to myself, I can really love you more.

It is time for me to let go of the old habits of thinking that I need to save, fix or protect you, *or* try to be whatever you want me to be. I need to really focus on my own passions and dreams. I really want to be true to myself. I want the freedom to do or be whatever I want to without fear that you will not like it, or that you will reject me.

If I am so afraid of you that I must repress my feelings, ideas or thoughts—or do everything you ask of me at the moment you want something, then I am in a co-dependent relationship with you. If I feel like nothing without you, I have a lot of work to do on myself!

And, if you feel less than me and need to be around me all the time to feel okay or safe or worthy, then you have a lot of work to do on yourself. And of course, if we are yelling at each other or hurting each other in any way, then there is a lot of work for both of us to do.

*The truth is, I really want to love you and connect deeply more and more. I just want our relationship to be healthy, and I do not want to be the one taking care of you nor do I want you to feel responsible for me.*

*In a healthy relationship, we both practice excellent self-care. We speak our truth, share our feelings, respond to each other in loving kindness, and know that we are safe—no matter what.*

I am open to this new way of living in relationship with you. Yes, I like it.

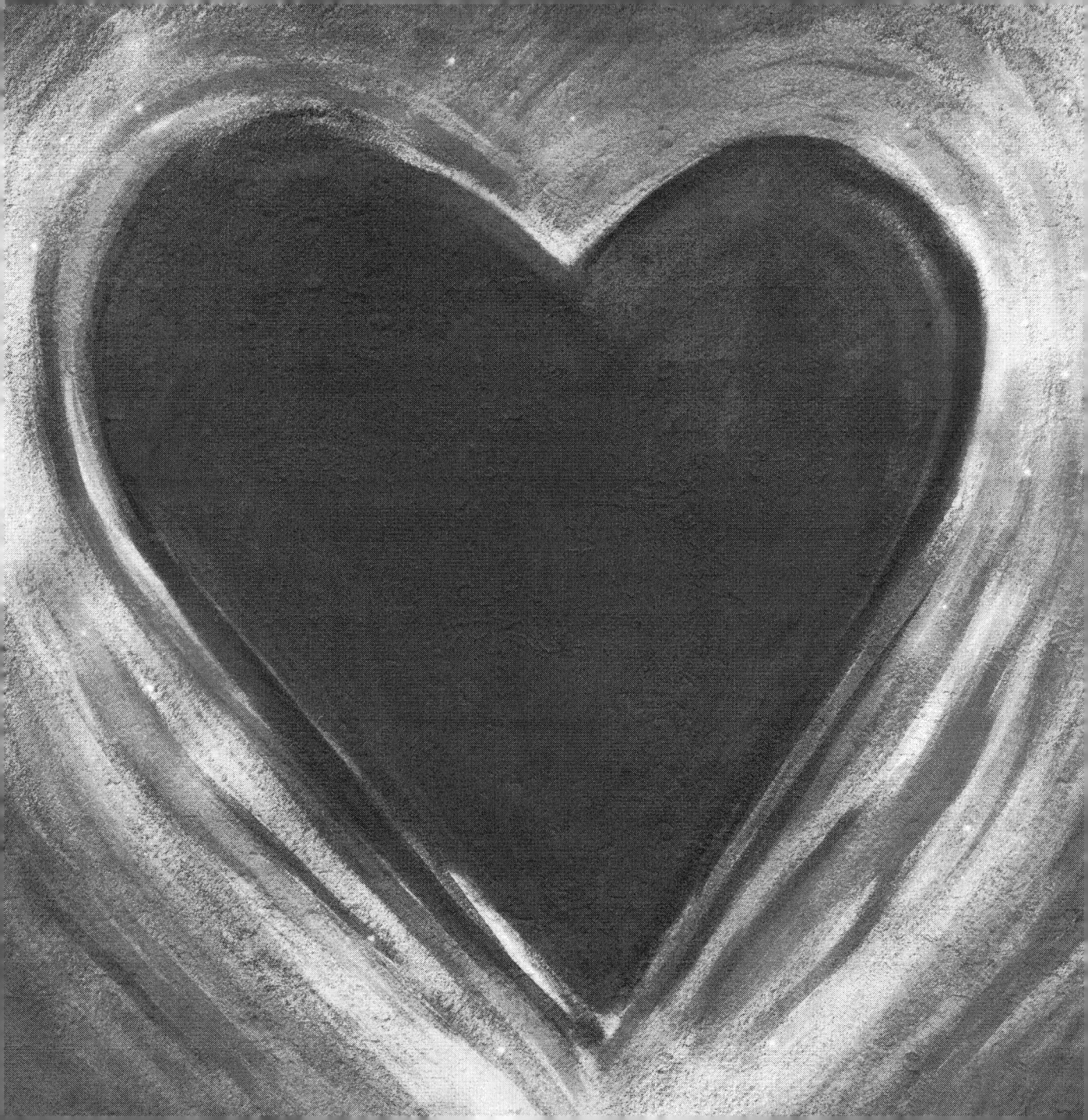

# CHAPTER TWO

Embracing Feelings

## Principle #8

Real emotional intimacy and real love is about two people who allow each other freedom, individuality, the right to be real and the right to feel.

Real love and true emotional intimacy exists when two people can be completely free to be real, whatever that means in the moment. Being real means that I have the freedom and safety to be who I am, to express who I am in the now according to me.

In order to discover the *real me*, I must take some time to explore everything I love. It is important for me to find my passion and power, to uncover all my parts, to bring to light what it is I came here to do on the earth. Perhaps I came here to be the best mother or father in the whole world... to raise children in loving kindness. Or perhaps I am supposed to be a rocket scientist or a musician or a career person. Whatever it is, I am here to do it, and it is part of my very core. If I do not discover who I am on the inside, I will not be able to love another human being fully. I will end up getting my needs met through other people with control, manipulation, martyrdom and victimhood. When I am me without guilt, I am free!

*I want to be real, authentic, genuine and true to myself. Sometimes I have to figure out what that really means.* Intimacy without Responsibility *means that I can love what I love, say what I want to say, be who I want to be, do what I want to do WITHOUT FEAR that you will not like it, or like me. And, I want to be able to do the same thing for you. It is okay that we do not like the same things.*

*I am committed to speaking my EMOTIONAL TRUTH. That means telling you how I really FEEL, who I really AM, what my ideas are. In this way, I am allowing myself to be vulnerable and genuine. I hope and wish that you can validate who I am, without telling me I should be or think or do or feel differently.*

## Principle #9

In order to be emotionally honest with you, I must express my feelings... instead of my opinions, judgements, defenses, explanations or helpful fixes and teachings.

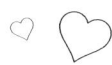

Most people just want to be real and be *validated* for however they feel, without judgement, criticism, or opinions. We all need to be *heard*. Our feelings need to be acknowledged.

When we are practicing *Intimacy without Responsibility*, we enjoy being able to express a feeling and have our significant other *just hear the feeling...* and *acknowledge* the feeling. That is all.

Feelings are energy in motion, vibrational signatures of the moment, chemical reactions in our body. They are not right or wrong. Some feelings are painful and some are joyful. When we hear our loved one's problems or feelings of pain it is natural to want to fix, teach them something, share our experience, explain ourselves, give opinions, etc. And this is not the first order of business in healthy loving communication.

The first step is just to validate and hear the feeling.

*When I am communicating with you, I am willing to hear your feelings. I am willing to hear your pain as well as your joy. And, I am willing just to hear you and say, "I hear you... I hear you are feeling _____."*

*You have the right to feel however you feel without me fixing you or telling you about me or telling you not to feel a certain way or giving you my opinion of the situation. And I ask you just to HEAR my feelings first without trying to fix me or tell me what I should do or give me your opinion or any of that stuff. Let's do that for each other, please. It is really nice to feel like I am seen and heard.*

# Principle #10

If I have a reaction to another person's expression of feelings, it is important for me *next* to express my own feeling, instead of defending or explaining myself.

When you are expressing your pain, so often I automatically want to tell you what to do to stop your pain. Or if your pain is about me, I may not hear you and I will begin to explain myself, or defend my actions or judge your feeling as wrong. In this way I have not heard you, and I have taken your pain personally. In essence, your feeling is causing me fear of some kind of loss.

Reactions are about our past, not our present. So when I am reacting to you in a painful or joyful way, it is really about me—even though it may appear that I am trying to help you.

*Intimacy without Responsibility* means that I honor your feelings, give you the right to feel pain about me or anything else… and become aware of how I feel because of it. Then, it is *my responsibility* to express how I feel… without defending.

Expressing feelings does not mean I am going to tell you what *I think*… a thought is an idea, a view, an opinion, conclusion or judgement. A feeling is a physical sensation in the body—an emotion—energy in motion. Basic feelings are mad, sad, happy, shame, guilt, fear, and love….

So, express like this: *I felt scared when you said you were mad. When you get mad it triggers my fear of anger. OR, I feel love when I see you crying and it makes me want to protect and fix you.*

*I am doing my best today to express my feelings, instead of my thoughts, and to be very aware of my REACTIONS, knowing that they are about my past, not you.*

# Principle #11

It is healthy and intimate to express anger in relationship. Anger is natural, normal and necessary to express in ways that are honoring.

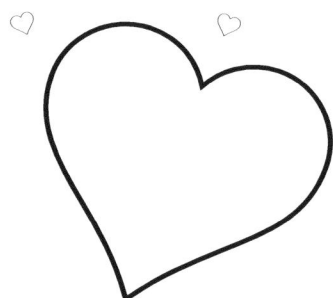

Anger is a very human emotion, and when expressed as it occurs, enhances intimacy in relationship. When two people take the risk to express their inner feelings or Self, they are pulled toward each other—and this is intimacy. When I am open and vulnerable and express my core feelings, I am taking responsibility for my own self and this is *Intimacy without Responsibility* for someone else.

It is normal to feel angry with people we love. Anger held inside becomes old and turns into resentment and even rage. If normal anger is not expressed when people live or work together, it merges with other feelings and creates personal walls and energy blockages.

*When I am practicing* Intimacy without Responsibility, *I feel free to tell you when I am angry. I can do this in a healthy way that honors us both, by asking you for some time to tell you about my feelings, instead of yelling or screaming or crying at some other time I am triggered. Speaking my truth about my anger is not always easy, because I may be afraid of my anger or afraid of your anger... or I may express anger with abusive words and actions, and this is not healthy either.*

*I am willing to understand that your being angry with me does not mean that you do not love me. Quite the opposite—when you tell me your truth, or I tell you my truth, we are opening up to our authentic and real selves in the moment, and that always pulls us closer together. We may not always agree on things, and I hope we don't because it would be boring always to think and believe and do the same thing. I am willing today to share my anger in a way that honors you and me.*

## Principle #12

I can give emotional love and support in a healthy way, teach you what I have learned, share my opinions and even my ideas for helping to fix a problem without responsibility or obligation.

There is a time when we can share ideas, opinions and even our judgements about issues. This time comes *after* we validate our partner's feelings. And this time comes *after* we ask if our opinion or ideas can be heard. Certainly, friends, lovers, spouses and family have certain commonalities that attracted them together in the first place. So, there is a time to share the *how* to do something, when one is open for it.

*Now that you have really validated my feelings by telling me what you heard me saying, and then responding to me, expressing your real feelings and reaction—I am able to hear your opinion or some solution to my problem. I may even want to hear your explanation about something that happened. However, please ask me first if I desire your input. I will honor you in this same way.*

*If you try to teach me first, I may not hear you, and I may even be resentful of you as the authority, trying to parent me, especially if I do not believe in myself or have low self worth. When you try to teach me or give me your opinion too soon, you are taking away my power to think for myself or solve my own problems. When you feel responsible or obligated to fix me, that is really about your need to fix... not about my need.*

*The time will come when I really do want your important information about a subject or your ideas about what I could do. And notice, I say COULD versus SHOULD… because should is a judgment and could is an opportunity.*

*I am committed to practicing this way of communication and I hope you will do the same for me.*

## Principle #13

My feelings are my truth. Your feelings are your truth. Our perceptions of everything come from our personal, unique filters and operating system.

Please honor my feelings and I will honor yours, even if I have a different opinion of what is happening or a different perception of what is happening.

Surely all of our perceptions or the way we interpret something will not be the same, because we grew up in different households. The way we filter and perceive the same event can really be different. We cannot tell people that they are right about a feeling or wrong about a feeling... feelings just happen, and they just are what they are.

*Intimacy without Responsibility* is a practice that lets go of having to be right, or of someone having to be wrong. In this work, we honor the fact that each person in a relationship comes with their own unique perception filters and operating system. This system is like the hard drive of a computer—and is not easy to change without re-programming. So, there is no reason to fight or give a lot of energy to *prove* you are right and someone is wrong. This most important principle is about honoring and being willing to listen to different perceptions as truth for whoever is communicating.

*I would like to ask you to honor my perception and really understand that I may have a different way of seeing things than you at times. I will do this for you, as well. Perhaps if we are very loving and open, we could invite each other to HEAR our different perceptions about something, which may or may not change the way we see that thing.*

*I am willing to change my perception if it makes sense to me, especially if I am actually re-acting in fear and anxiety and desire peace and calm.*

## Principle #14

I face my fears of intimacy and embrace all my feelings,
knowing that my feelings create my reality.
Whatever I am feeling about our relationship, I am creating.

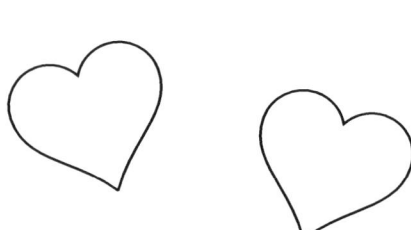

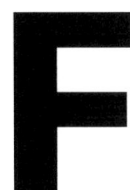ear is the core feeling under many painful emotions or low vibrational feelings. Other fear based feelings include anger, hate, guilt, resentment, need for approval, overwhelmed burden, depression, revenge, blame, powerlessness and shame.

It is important to release low vibrational feelings inside, in order to practice *Intimacy without Responsibility*—so that you can truly love without fear. It is important to clear out any of the negative and painful emotions that your body holds onto on a regular basis to be free.

When someone lives in fear, they usually blame others for life experiences and painful communication as well as project their own shame and fear on others through judgement, anger, name-calling and put-downs. This is sad.

*If and when I am holding onto fear-based feelings about you, or myself, I am not free. I commit to examining any fears I have that have been repressed, because they will affect all my thoughts, opinions, judgments and feelings about you and whatever you are doing or saying.*

*I do not want to project my fear, or anger, guilt or shame on you. And I do not want you to project on me either. I commit to staying clear and doing whatever it is I need to do, to release feelings of fear.*

*As I take the risk to move through old pain, I can let go and move into a higher and higher vibration and walk into my power! As I take care of myself, heal and love myself, I can love you more deeply because I will not be afraid.*

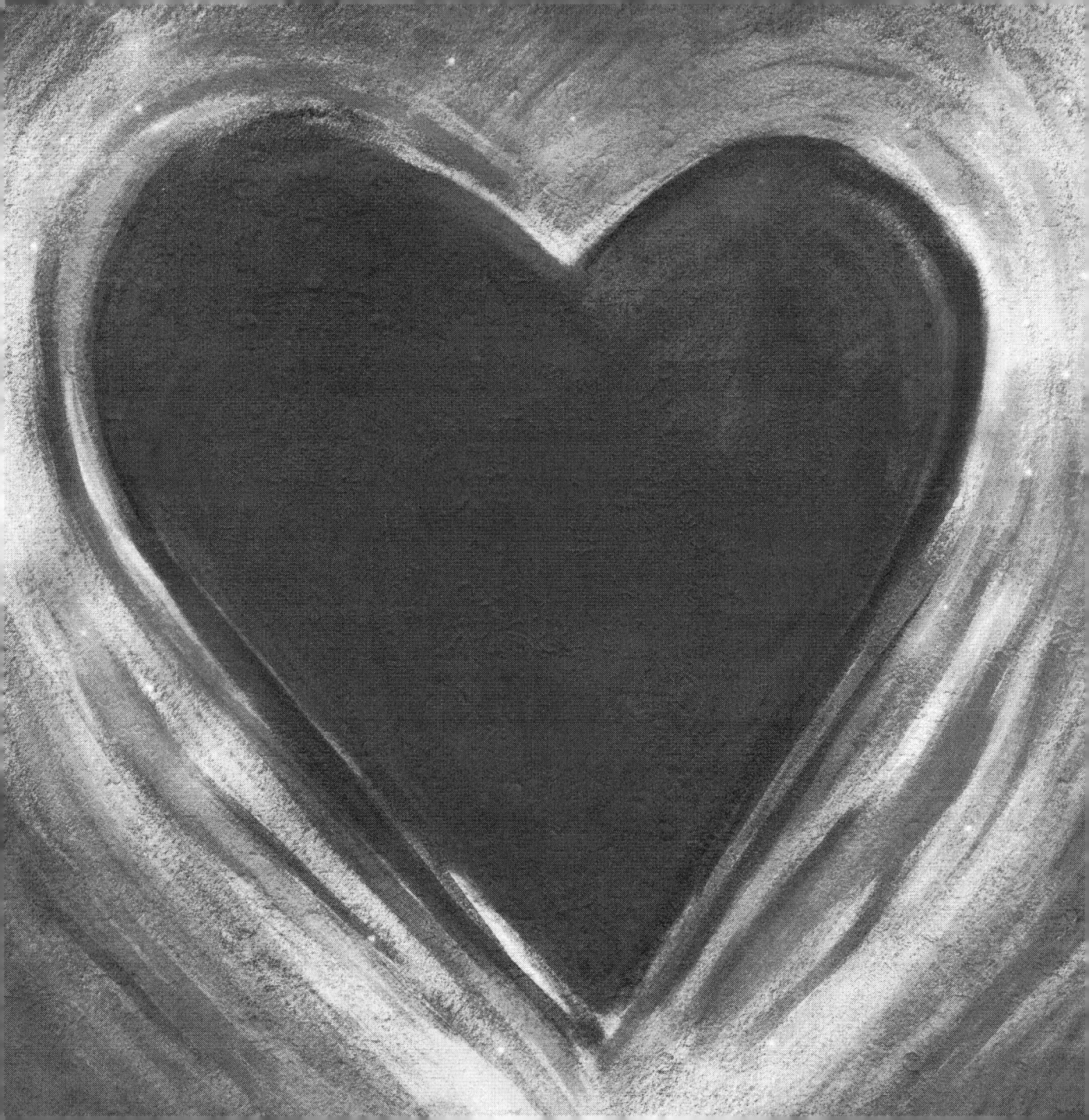

# CHAPTER THREE

Wound Re-Enactments

## Principle #15

All my life experiences translate into what is now my present belief system and core issues that live inside me.

My body remembers everything—especially old wounds, which eventually get re-enacted in my relationship.

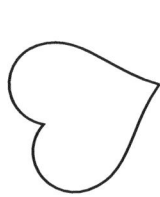 

Brain studies reveal that we have three brains connected closely together, each embodying a different stage of human evolution. The old brain (the medulla and the spinal cord) is called our reptilian brain and governs our survival instincts, like food, shelter, mating/sex, protection/defense and our habits. Above this area is the limbic system or the old mammalian brain, which is the seat of our emotions—processing and receiving stimulation/input, then communicating with other layers of our brain. The third brain is called the new mammalian brain or the neocortex that is our thinking brain controlling abstract reasoning.

The limbic system is the part of our brain that holds our emotions and any painful life experiences with a mechanism or gate that stops us from conscious awareness of our pain.

*Subconscious pain becomes a dominant aspect of my personality without me knowing it. And that dominant part of my psyche becomes the foundation for all my beliefs about life, people, love, marriage, relationship, children, etc. My inner pain becomes the filter through which I see everything with resulting thoughts and feelings that match it. Feelings are the vibrational energy that magnetize people, places and things into my life, giving me all the experiences I have had.*

*My un-expressed, subconscious wounds become re-enacted with the people around me, especially you, because I want to love you and I want you to love me in a way that really works well. I commit myself now to discovering whatever is in my subconscious... no matter what or how long it takes.*

## Principle #16

My conception, womb, birth and early childhood experiences become a part of my relationship with you.

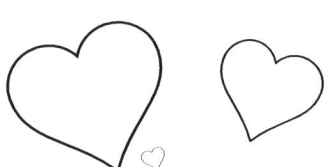

Your first life imprint/blueprint is your womb and birth experience—an imprint or pattern that gets re-enacted over and over again in your life. If you notice carfully, you will see that your early childhood experiences interestingly match your birth process – and then you attract relationships and people into your life who resemble your birth and early experiences. We call this *wound re-enactment!*

It is valuable in the healing work to gather information about your birth so to understand these patterns. Although you are not conscious of your birth and do not remember it, your body remembers exactly how you were born. Know this: You will live your life and experience relationship the way you were born! This also holds true for everything else that happened after birth, especially the first six years of childhood, as these are the imprinting years.

*The life experiences I had with my mother, father, siblings, teachers and other adults created my belief system about love, safety, vulnerability, care-taking, power, marriage, communication, and all the important subjects I need to feel positive and powerful about, in order to have and experience real love.*

*Relationship and intimacy issues are all about wound re-enactment. Sooner or later, my unresolved core issues will surface with the person or people I am in relationship with. The good news is that I can reverse the patterns and heal my past at the same time. It is all good. I am committed to healing and transforming any belief, pattern, thought or feeling that gets in the way of my having healthy and loving relationships.*

# Principle #17

At the moment of my birth, I take on core beliefs that effect my interpretation of everything in my life.

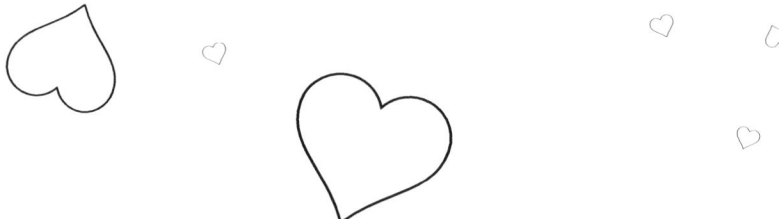

The mere pressure of fitting a head through a small opening is traumatic in itself, therefore, all of us have some kind of birth trauma and birth imprint, resulting in decisions and beliefs we made at that moment, effecting everything we do, including how we are in relationship, who and what we attract into our lives.

Children whose mothers were given drugs during birth may, as adults, rely on drugs or some kind of substance to "get through things," numbing themselves when there is fear or pain, real or imagined. In relationship, someone with this birth pattern may become overwhelmed, unable to communicate or get through an issue and may develop addictions that further complicate relationship with a core belief of—*I need this to get through.*

Children, who had the umbilical cord wrapped around their neck at birth, may find themselves "choking" in life in various ways or having many problems with sore throats or breathing. In relationship, this person may feel that a significant other is a *pain in the neck or choking out their life force!*

A baby may be pulled out of the birth canal by forceps or a doctor who hung them upside down and spanked them, a common practice in the old days. This baby may come to believe that doctors or *men or women hurt them.*

*Eventually, I unconsciously set up situations with my loved one to reinforce and re-enact my original beliefs and decisions. I am therefore committed to revealing and healing my original birth pattern so that it no longer needs to be acted out in the present.*

# Principle #18

Any issues or pain I have not resolved with my parents will become re-enacted with you... like my unresolved old wounds or trauma, something I lost, something I always needed or something I do not even know.

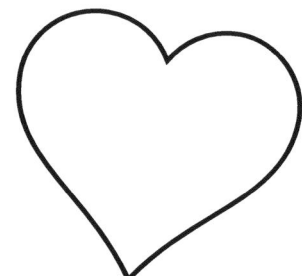
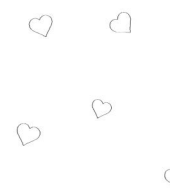

It is important to realize that any unresolved issues I have with my parents will come up in my relationships. If I do not heal, transform and integrate the negative or painful experiences that occurred between me and my parents, my love relationship will not work and I will be unable to practice *Intimacy without Responsibility*.

Any unfinished business from my past will always come up for me with others because I will unconsciously attract it. I will always attract and recreate situations that mirror my original pain, until they are resolved, because I will always attract that which is familiar to me. Anything that has anything to do with love brings up anything unlike love first.

*Any pain or fear I have not remembered or faced, any place I hold judgment, resentment, hate, guilt, fear, anger or anything I lost or always needed will come up for healing through relationships. Although possibly thought of as bad news, this is really good news! Because, once I really get this principle, I am able to embrace my feelings and whatever dynamics are occurring in my relationships in a way that gives me a starting point for transformation. Instead of blaming someone else, leaving or running away from the situation, I am able to understand what has unconsciously occurred and work on a resolution. WOW! I see that eventually, similar dynamicas and experiences will be re- created until the original pain is resolved.*

*I am willing and able to face my fears about all of this, being open to my own healing, transformation and truth about my early relationship with my parents. Eventually, as I resolve the issues inside me, I will no longer fear love or re-enact the original pain.*

## Principle #19

Whenever I have a problem or issue with you, I have an opportunity to heal and transform something inside me.

Our issues dysfunctionally fit together like puzzle pieces.

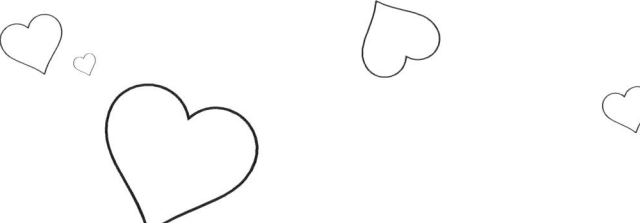

When my mind is open and I embrace these principles, I begin to realize that all my problems and issues are really opportunities to heal myself!

If I have a core issue of abandonment, you probably have a core issue of enmeshment. If I have a core issue of care-taking my parents from an early age, I will attract a partner who needs to be taken care of, too (or at least I think I have to). If my father was an alcoholic, I will surely attract another alcoholic or someone with addiction problems. If my mother had an affair with someone, then I will attract someone who does the same (or at least I will fear that this will happen to me). If my father was a rage-aholic, yelling, hitting and putting me down, I will attract a mate who may do the same, or if he even raises his voice, I will say he is abusing me.

Examples of core issues are: abandonment, alcoholism and addiction, death, loss, poverty, neglect, sexual abuse, physical abuse, emotional abuse, religious abuse, illness of family members, codependency and care-taking, and the many core issues from womb and birth.

*I am learning that my core issues get re-enacted in my relationship with you, and the same is happening for you.*

*I am committed to clarity and discovery of my own core issues, and then healing, transforming and reversing the issue or belief that stops me from having a close, loving and intimate relationship with you.*

# Principle #20

Every relationship I have is mirroring something about me that is wanting to come up into consciousness for my healing and transformation... for my wholeness and the evolution of my soul.

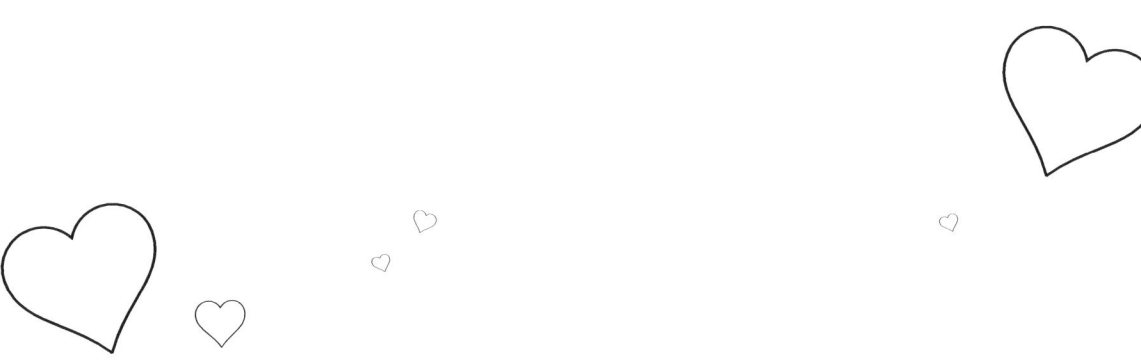

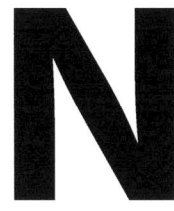ow it is time to realize that all relationships are *mirroring* something back to you about yourself. It does not matter if that something about you is painful or joyful, positive or negative… the *mirror* goes both ways, as does a real mirror. If I look in a mirror, the image is *me* at that moment, no matter if I look good or not!

Because of this principle, we can now say that *there is never a reason to blame anyone for doing something to you. Most* people are acting out their own subconscious core issues, beliefs, thoughts and feelings, and are motivated by their own past and present experiences stored in the body/mind. *Most* people do not set out to have a bad or painful experience and do not consciously plan to hurt someone else. Most people just want to love and be loved and important to someone else.

*My painful or joyful experiences with you are literally and energetically MATCHING a similar wave frequency in me. Sometimes the mirroring back is joyful and sometimes it is painful. AND this pain can assist me in realizing that it is matching something in me or something STILL in me (even through I have done much healing work) that I need to work on next. And I will.*

*Thank you for being my greatest teacher. The pain I have felt because of your behavior is opening me up to remembering my original core wound, so that I can heal it and never have to go through this experience again.*

# Principle #21

Whatever is going on between you and me right now (painful or joyful) is happening for a powerful purpose.

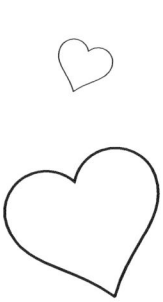

*I am learning how to be close to you without taking responsibility for your feelings, actions, behaviors, beliefs or thoughts. That is really freedom. I can be who I am, and you can be who you are. I do not have to try to change you, manipulate situations, control things or fix anything about you or your life. I can just BE and let you BE who you are, having the consequences and results that just happen. And I choose to believe everything is happening and moving toward wholeness and the highest good, even when it does not feel like it.*

*In order for you to become all you are meant to be, I must let go of wanting you to do something a certain way. When I try to force you to do something my way or see something from my perception, I am only attracting resistance, because you will always mirror back the same energy that I am putting out or that is stored in my body.*

*Whatever is going on between you and me right now is happening for a powerful purpose. Somehow, somewhere—before we came to this earth in our human form, we decided to have these experiences, so our souls could evolve. So, everything that is happening is very powerful and wonderful, even if it feels hard and challenging, painful and crazy.*

*I love myself and I love you. Thank you for going through all this pain with me. Thank you for going through all this joy with me. I love learning how to take care of myself and be intimate with you, too. I am alive and free. By the way, I let go of our agreement to unconsciously create this pain together. I am ready to have a new experience in my life with you.*

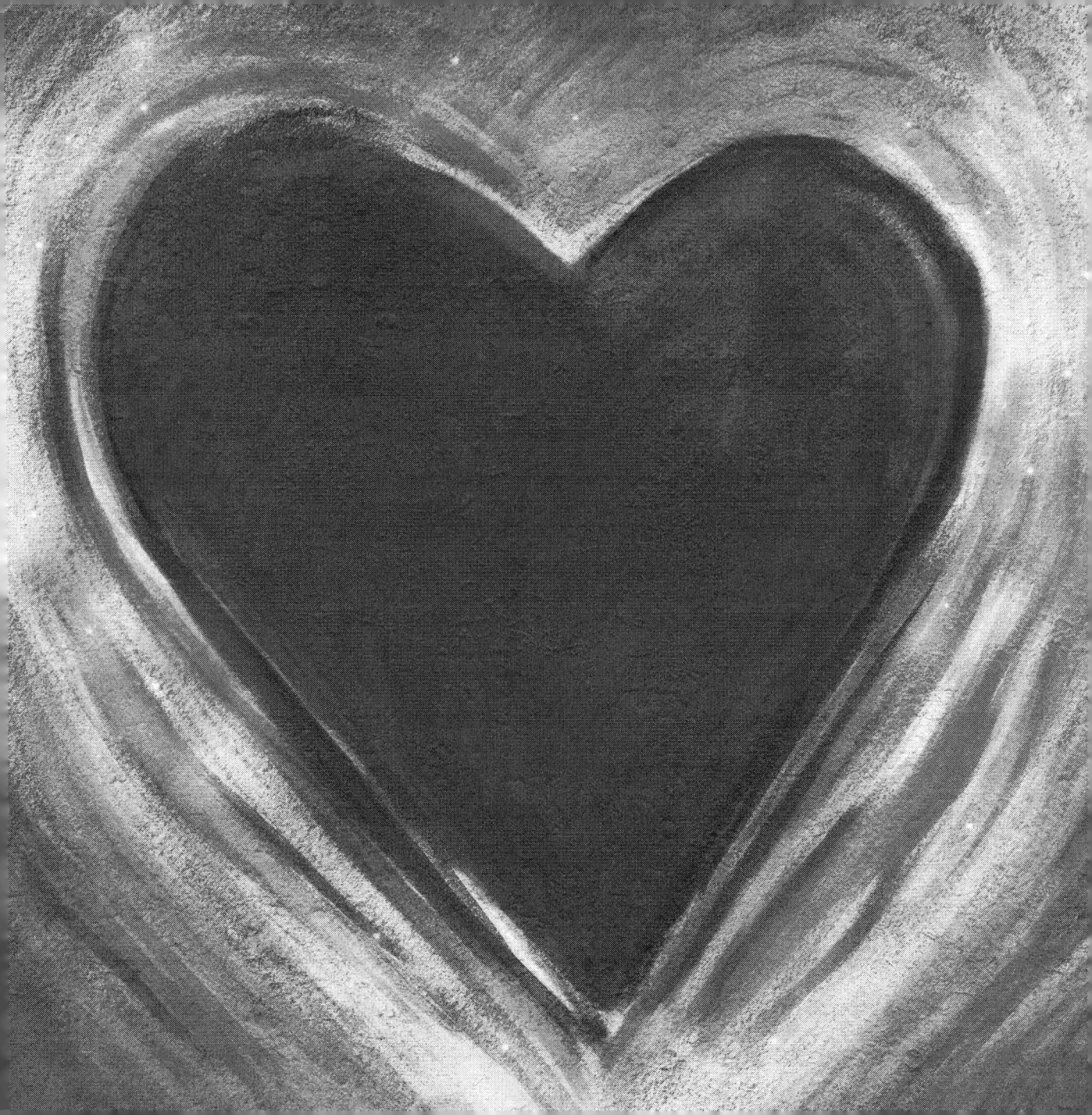

# CHAPTER FOUR

Intimacy Boundaries

# Principle #22

I have the right to have my own personal space and boundaries to create reasonable limits and guidelines for others.

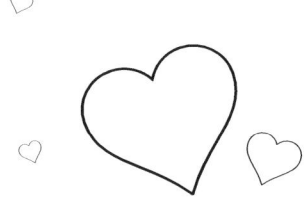

Closely related to wound re-enactment and core issues is the topic of personal, psychological and physical boundaries. It is healthy to decide what I need in the way of psychological and personal space, so I can feel safe in my world and with you. So, I have certain limits!

Issues of personal space and boundaries are big for those who have had physical, sexual, and emotional abuse—violations of personal space during childhood, the damaged amygdala in the brain becoming strongly activated when people get physically close.

People practicing *Intimacy without Responsibility,* or any two people who desire to have a loving, lasting and successful relationship, need a clear sense of Self—a personal identity and high self-esteem to be able to create healthy boundaries and respect boundaries set by a significant other.

We do the healing work on our core issues and dysfunctional personal patterns, in order to create new neural pathways in the brain. This enables us to be personally strong and powerful, so that we can communicate without taking things personally and set healthy personal boundaries.

*I desire to understand my core issues and reactions to you more and more deeply. I am committed to healing whatever it is that keeps me in the same old reaction patterns with you. I commit also to creating my own personal boundaries for Self—and I will do everything I can to decide what I will do if and when you step outside of my limits. In this way, I am loving myself, keeping myself safe as well as honoring our relationship.*

## Principle #23

I can love deeply and still have a need for my own personal space. I honor your needs for space, as well, and will not take it personally if you need more space than I do.

Some people need more personal space than others, a unique and individual decision and personal character choice. Those who were raised in large families without a lot of space, those whose personal space was invaded by abuse or aggression, those who were engulfed or enmeshed by parents, those who truly did not have a safe space to find peace, those who took on the emotional needs of parents, siblings or other people, and even those who were in the womb or birth canal for a long time really seem to need and desire *space* (more than others), fearing closeness and intimacy.

People who were left alone in large spaces, those who felt abandoned and unloved, those who needed connection and touch, those whose space was not invaded by abuse or aggression may *not* desire *space* in relationship in the same way. In fact, this person may need an abundance of touch to feel loved.

Our spatial needs and feelings have everything to do with whatever happened to us from the moment of conception. There is no right or wrong about our spatial feelings and needs. Those who do need more space fear intimacy and need space and freedom in relationship. This includes sexual intimacy as well as emotional intimacy.

Often in relationship, one person needs space and is fearful of closeness, and the other needs closeness and is fearful of space! When this happens, it is all part of a perfect process and an opportunity for healing. *I am willing to understand and not take it personally if you need more space than I do, and I ask you to do the same for me.*

## Principle #24

I am committed to understanding my own boundary issues, knowing I must do so to practice *Intimacy without Responsibility*.

According to Nina Brown, EdD, LPC, NCC, there are four types of psychological boundaries:

**Soft:** A person with soft boundaries merges with other people's boundaries. Someone with a soft boundary is easily manipulated.

**Spongy:** A person with spongy boundaries is like a combination of having soft and rigid boundaries. They permit less emotional contagion than soft boundaries but more than rigid. People with spongy boundaries are unsure what to let in and what to keep out.

**Rigid:** A person with rigid boundaries is closed or walled off so nobody can get close to them either physically or emotionally. This is often the case if someone has been physically, emotionally, or psychologically abused. Rigid boundaries can be selective which depend on time, place or circumstances and are usually based on a bad previous experience in a similar situation.

**Flexible:** This is the ideal. Similar to selective rigid boundaries but the person has more control. The person decides what to let in and what to keep out, are resistant to emotional contagion, manipulation and are difficult to exploit.

*I am getting more and more clear about my own boundaries. I have been so soft in my boundaries with loved ones. I am committed to facing my fears and setting boundaries, especially with those who do not respect mine.*

# Principle #25

I am ready to decide and select *what and whom* to let in and keep out of my life, so that I can experience healthy boundaries.

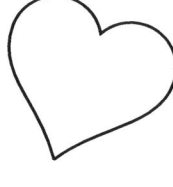

So it seems that *flexible* boundaries are ideal. When I have flexible boundaries, I am able to be selective about who or what I allow into my life and relationships. I do not want to merge with someone else and have *soft* or enmeshed boundaries, not knowing the difference between us. I do not want *spongy* boundaries where I am confused and do not know who or what to let in my life—being wishy-washy. And I do not want to be physically or emotionally closed off from others either, with *rigid* boundaries—or I will never experience true love and intimacy (without responsibility.)

Of course, I do not want to be manipulated, exploited or susceptible to emotional contagion. And I do not want to do this to others either.

*I am ready to set limits to protect myself from being manipulated or enmeshed with the emotional needs of others. I desire to separate my thoughts and feelings from others and take responsibility for what I am doing, thinking, feeling and being.*

*I am ready to be a full adult on my own. I am ready to face my fears about setting boundaries, ask for help in understanding them, and be willing to take the risk to tell and share them with others in my life. I will learn how to be close to you without trying to control or manipulate you. I ask that you do the same. I will learn how to be close to you without being enmeshed with you. Please do this for me as well. I will be flexible, so we can be close, yet sometimes I may have to keep a distance to protect myself physically or emotionally. I will honor your wish, if you need to do the same. And, I commit to doing my work on me, so it will all be easier.*

## Principle #26

I am practicing *Intimacy without Responsibility,* as I become interdependent, rather than dependent or independent.

The goal is to become *interdependent* (flexible, open, healthy) in relationship, rather than dependent (needy) or independent. *Intimacy without Responsibility* is really about learning what real true intimacy can be like. When you have good, healthy, flexible boundaries, you are taking care of your own Self first with the ability to be to give and receive.

When you are interdependent, you have a strong relationship with your Self and will not feel threatened by intimacy with others or by your partner's special qualities, successes, uniqueness or anything else. Nor will you feel threatened when your partner does not want to be with you all the time—requesting personal space. It is healthy to have your own time, space, things, rooms, friends, passions and interests! And it is wonderful when you have time, space, things, rooms, friends, passions and interests together, too.

One who is interdependent respects the fact that a partner or loved one is different from them—with their own personal perceptions, feelings, thoughts, beliefs, opinions and personal boundaries. Differences are respected in one who is interdependent and flexible. This is really a core principle of this work and opens people to incredibly rich, genuine, happy and fulfilling personal and love relationships.

*I am ready to be interdependent in all ways. I am ready to fully respect my Self, to be flexible and open making good choices about what I will allow in my life from now on. I let go of any kind of judgment, manipulation or belief that you should be like me. I honor that you are as you are, AND that may or may not fit within my healthy boundaries. We shall see....*

## Principle #27

I am committed to improving my Self-worth and reversing dysfunctional codependent behavior patterns as a necessary part of the ability to practice *Intimacy without Responsibility*.

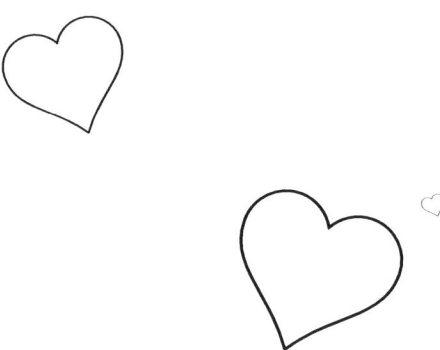

When I do not love myself and do not know who I am, I do not have my own identity and then I will not have healthy boundaries. If I do not feel worthy or good enough, I may tend to get my identity from you in some way—just like when I was a little child. Then, when this happens, I become the child, and you become the parent, and our relationship is not equal.

Or, if in my family of origin, I had to become a surrogate spouse to my mother or father—or the family hero to keep everything balanced and safe—I will take on that kind of role in my love relationships. I will be the parent and treat my significant other or even people in general as children and our relationship is not equal.

These kinds of patterns are co-dependent, dysfunctional and painful. And I am so accustomed to living this way that I often do not realize what I am doing or how I am with other people. At times, I do not even know who I am without the problems, drama and roles I have played. Who am I? And what do I really want? Am I still a child in some relationships, or am I parenting an adult? I want to be whole and fulfilled by myself. I want a life without dysfunctional and codependent patterns being re-enacted.

*Today, I am willing to do whatever it takes to love myself and reverse dysfunctional behavior patterns that live in me, even it means that I must say goodbye to someone or not take care of you anymore, or give up some kind of security I get from you. I may even have to move, surrender my job or change something big... just to take care of my Self, become whole, and improve my self-worth. I can and I will!*

## Principle #28

I am willing now to give myself permission to be who I am, ask for what I want, settle for nothing but the greatest and best for myself and to have healthy boundaries.

*I deserve the best, and I am no longer willing to say that I am going to keep things the way they are, just so I do not upset the apple cart! I am ready to explore everything life has to offer, and I am setting new boundaries.*

*I will not give up the chance to be the person I was meant to be, and I am not willing to give up my dreams just so that YOU do not feel less than me. I will not give up myself just to have the security of being with you. That will not work anymore. We are equal. I will not feel less than—or more superior to—you or anyone, and I will not settle for a mediocre life or relationship.*

*We can both do well in our lives, make money, have friends, and live to our highest potential. It is not my job to support you when you have the ability to do things for yourself. It is time for me to TRUST you in all ways, and it is time for you to TRUST me in all ways, if our relationship is to be fulfilling.*

*I let go of feeling guilty if I am happy and you are not happy! We are both responsible for creating our own happiness. I may not always be available to you when you want or need me. And I am aware that you may not always be available to me when I want or need you. I will support your dreams and I allow you to have your life experiences even if this means you experience pain or failure of some kind. I am letting go of rescuing you. Please treat me with respect and love. It is not okay with me to be in relationship with someone who abuses me in any way. I will have to say goodbye if that happens. And please do your own healing work. I have decided that I do not want to be in relationship with anyone who is not consciously working on personal growth.*

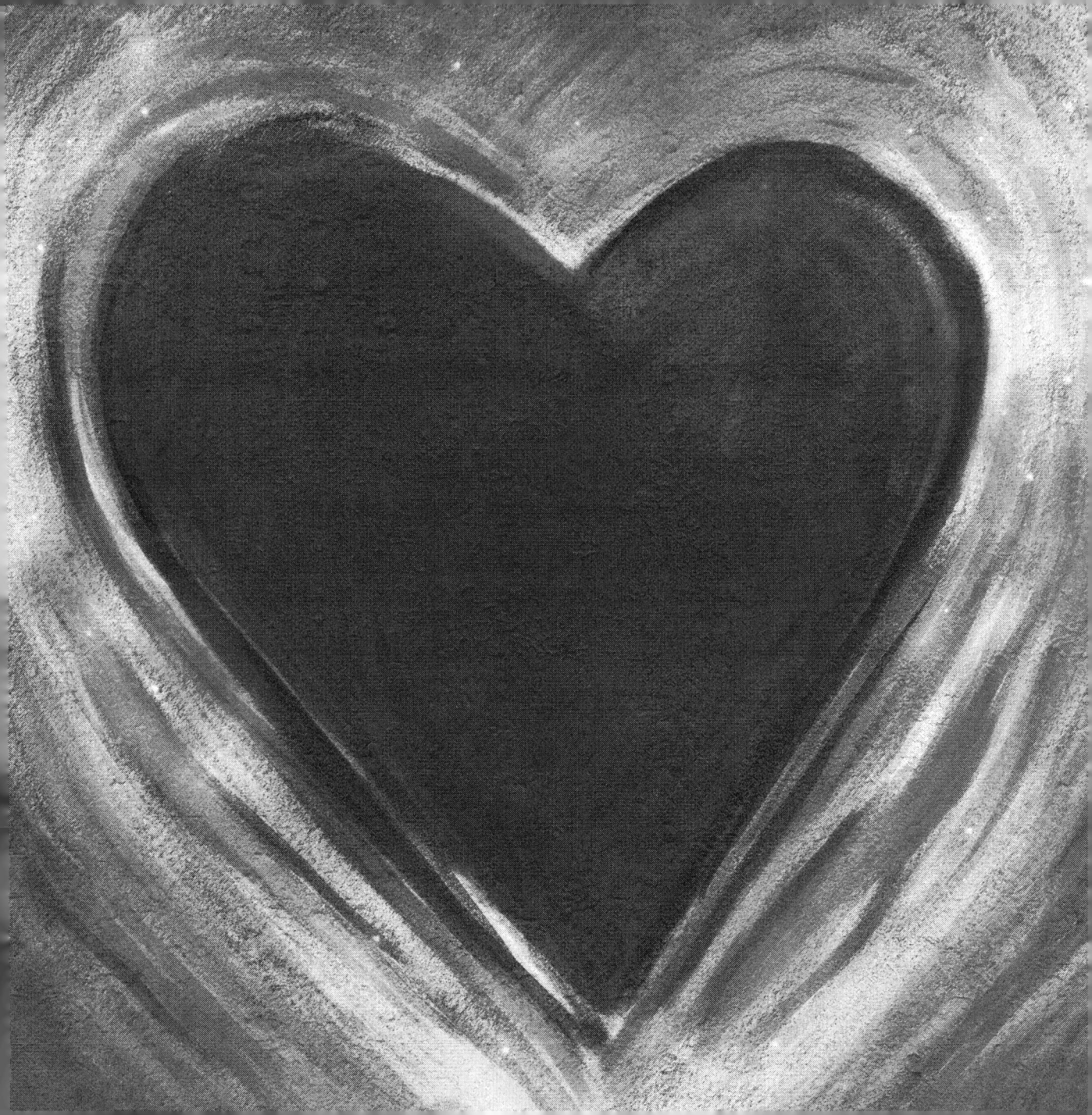

# CHAPTER FIVE

Responsibility vs. Blame

# Principle #29

I never again need to blame you or even *me* for problems in our relationship. Instead, I will take responsibility for my creations.

**I**ntimacy without Responsibility adheres to the *No Blame* principle. If you blame your partner for what he or she is doing to you, you will not heal. As long as you are blaming another person, you are a victim. Instead, it is important to think, "I have re-created my past feelings and negative beliefs about myself. When I was young, my dad left me and I begged him not to go. So, now I think you are going to leave too, and then I *react*."

And next, you think, "My reaction and feeling was based on my old belief system that dad will leave and he must not love me or want me… and this situation feels similar. *I have attracted* this situation *so that I can heal the original pain!* What a wonderful thing!"

*This work is about taking 100% responsibility for what it is that I am experiencing in my life and in my relationship challenges. This time, instead of reacting the same old way, re-living the pattern over and over, I am willing to take responsibility for my creation. In so doing, I am not blaming myself either. My soul has assisted me in re-creating a similar experience, so I can heal. In truth, this all means that I am moving toward wholeness.*

*I choose now to perceive my life from this viewpoint. In this way, I never again need to blame anyone for anything. This does not mean that I will never feel angry or resentful or scared… and I may react again. The thing is—I will PROCESS the experience through and apply this powerful way of being with it.*

## Principle #30

As I continue to work on my own wholeness, I know that your feelings, opinions and judgements are about you, not me. I will, therefore, do everything I can not to take things personally.

**B**ecause I know that everything happening is a way my soul is assisting me in moving toward wholeness, I choose not to take any of your painful feelings, opinions, judgments or behaviors personally. Your feelings and thoughts are about you, mine are about me.

*But I do take them personally at times, sometimes… a lot! OK. So, it is time to become aware of this principle, and do my best to re-think, re-frame, re-vision, and re-image EVERYTHING that I seem to take personally.*

What if …. *everything* in the whole world was really a reflection of *you*. What if everything you see, hear, taste, smell, experience—painful or joyful—is really *you* looking back at *you*—a giant mirror always. And that mirror is really just an incredible way for you to discover the mysteries of yourself, the unconscious, repressed information that lives inside your body/mind. I think it's true.

You are here for a reason. There are no mistakes. Every experience is matching your own energy inside. So, as you change your own energy, you have a new experience. You are hearing and learning this information now, because you are ready to really heal your life.

*When I realize that my world perfectly reflects whatever is inside me (as above, so below), I then have incredible power at my fingertips... power to be 100% responsible for my experiences. As I heal my original pain, I no longer need to blame you or anyone else. We are all a part of the creation.*

## Principle #31

As I continue to learn and embrace these principles, I am free.
I discover that everything is happening for a reason,
and I am right on schedule.

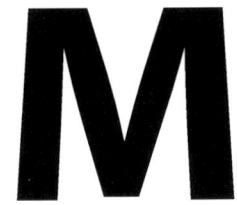any have been living uninformed, in a prison of fear, denying self expression—in doubt, confused, feeling separated from the very energy that created the universe. I can change my reality as I change my belief system, as I change my perception. I am that I am that I am.

Because you learned everything that you are doing, thinking, feeling, being, you can relearn. You can reprogram all old toxic messages that you came to believe about yourself or about love (that do not work.) Communication patterns and ways of seeing and being with your significant others were imprinted during your womb, birth and early childhood years.

*I know that I am right on schedule with my issues and experiences. I could not have done this or learned it any earlier—nor could anyone else. My old pain and old ways of perceiving has come to a place that desires change. The universe moves in cycles of death and re-birth—and that is what is happening to me now. I am dying to my old way of being with you in relationship. I am going through a natural cycle of change, just like the change of seasons in nature.*

*When I really embrace these principles and this work on Self, I am free. I am free to love someone without taking responsibility for him or her. I am free to experience pain and not blame anyone—and not blame myself for problems. I am free to be real and free to express everything inside me. I can look at problems in a way that empowers me rather than keeps me victimized by society or someone else. I realize I am just in my own personal relationship cycle, having started at the beginning, moving through the middle on to the end... real love.*

## Principle #32

If I am blaming you for something, I am choosing to be a victim... *victim consciousness* meaning that I have given up my power. When I am a victim, I give up responsibility for my manifestations.

**B**elow are common conscious and unconscious messages learned from family of origin, teachers, society, religion and authority figures. They support the notion of victim consciousness in relationship.

*Victim consciousness* is the belief that someone else has done something to you that is bad or unacceptable, and as a result, it is someone else's fault or responsibility that you are not happy.

- Something wrong has happened.
- I blame you for doing this or being that way.
- I judge the things you do and how you do them.
- I use the past to prove I am right and you are wrong.
- It is not okay that you are imperfect. I expect more of you.
- The facts are the facts. You have done something wrong.
- I resent you forever. I may forgive you, but I will never forget.
- You and I are separate.
- Something wrong or bad has happened. I suppose I could accept that.
- I guess I am just unlucky with relationships and life.
- Next time, I will be more in control of myself.
- Men/Women are all that way.
- Why me? Why does this always happen to me?
- Watch out! The world is not safe.

*I am willing to take responsibility for anything I did or did not do that hurt you, and I hope you are, too. At the same time, I will not blame either of us because it is all part of our process.*

## Principle #33

I choose to be the master... of my own core issues, core beliefs, thoughts, feelings and creations. I decide now to be the architect of my own life.

Here is a chart about RELATIONSHIP CYCLES. Notice that with the first two cycles, you are unconsciously unconscious… (not knowing what you did not know) reacting out of self-preservation and survival, even when it is joyful! In the middle of the cycle, you begin to become consciously unconscious (learning what you did not know) and applying it for healing and transformation, and finally you are unconsciously conscious (as it all becomes second nature now… *and you feel real true love*, which is the same as *Intimacy without Responsibility!*

| Primal Consciousness I | Primal Consciousness II | Higher Consciousness I | Higher Consciousness II | Transpersonal Consciousness |
|---|---|---|---|---|
| **Unconsciously Unconscious** | **Unconsciously Unconscious** | **Consciously Unconscious** | **Consciously Unconscious** | **Unconsciously Conscious** |
| Self Preservation | Self Preservation | Healing | Transformation | Transcendence |
| Romantic Love | Struggle | Awareness | Awakening | True Love |
| Attachment | Change | KNOWLEDGE Self Partner Core Issues Patterns Fear and Pain | TRANSMUTATION Re-framing Re-visioning Re-solving Re-member | COMPLETION Unconditional Giving and Receiving |
| Attraction | Frustration | | | |
| Illusion | Disillusionment | | | |
| Excitement | Anger, Fear, Panic | COMMITTMENT Personal Healing Partner Healing Risk Goals Intentions Relationship Principles | COMMUNICATION Feelings Validating Empathizing Mirroring | Intimacy without Responsibility or Obligation |
| Ecstasy/Oceanic | | | | |
| Desire | Pressure, control | | | Empathetic Loving Non Defensive |
| Joyful Transference | Painful Transference | | AWAKENING Inspiration Intuition Universal Truths Shadow | Spiritual Intimacy Synergy Joy |
| Grof's Birth Matrix I | Stuck/Impasse | Grof's Birth Matrix III | | |
| | Grof's Birth Matrix II | | Grof's Birth Matrix III | Grof's Birth Matrix IV |
| **Reaction** | **Reaction** | **Reaction/Response** | **Response** | **Spontaneity** |

## Principle #34

As I take responsibility for my own experiences—knowing I have attracted people and situations that match my inner Self at some level—I heal and change my inner Self. Then I have new experiences, and I may choose to change my life. When I take responsibility for all my experiences, I am free.

Finally it is time to answer the question that many are wondering about now. What about the people who really did hurt me, or raped someone, or hurt a child? Certainly, a little child has no power or understanding of all this. Did I attract that person into my life to have such a horrible experience? Or what if someone really is cheating on me, or hitting me, or will not pay attention to me or is an alcoholic or emotionally unavailable? Or what if I am the alcoholic or rage-addict or the one hurting others? Am I supposed just to say I am right on schedule and ignore this... that it is just karma?

*NO. Taking responsibility for my creations only means that I understand that my painful experiences are matching something inside me of the same vibrational frequency. The energy in the universe is attracted toward me like a radio signal to a chosen station. NO. Taking responsibility for my creations does not mean that I ignore, do not confront, or make excuses for people who hurt me or for my own behavior. NO. Healthy boundaries are part of the formula for healing. And, EXPRESSING my human feelings about what has happened to me is even more important. Likewise, I must take responsibility for any of my own behaviors or actions that have hurt someone else. So, the answer is NO... I will not ignore harmful behavior in myself or others.*

*It does mean… that I know this person or abuser is matching some part of my soul that holds the same kind of energy... like past wounds that are similar. (Or karma?) And I do know that if I realize this, take powerful action to discover and heal my own wounds, these kinds of experiences will stop.*

*Whenever I need to remember that I do not want to be a victim, I like to say this powerful phrase, "I wonder what this experience is matching in me... that I am ready to heal."*

## Principle #35

I am committed to speaking a language of power, communicating in loving kindness... and fighting fairly with you.

In order to practice *Intimacy without Responsibility* and Responsibility vs. Blame, it is important to commit to a language of power, which includes communicating in loving kindness and fair fighting without blame!

Here are the basics:

- Be 100% responsible for what you are creating…no blame.
- Rather than criticize, give opinions or lecture, ask your partner if an opinion is desired.
- Be assertive rather than passive or aggressive.
- Let go of judgment. Use the feelings formula.
- Speak to your partner with *"I"* statements rather that *"you"* statements.
- Talk about one thing at a time, and stay in the present moment. Do you best to *respond* versus *react*. Reaction means and *old* button is being pushed…(family of origin pain).
- Communicate *feelings* (process) rather that *details* (content).
- Honor the fact that both of you have different perceptions of the same event, which is true for each person. Loving kindness is not about having to be right or wrong.
- If you discover that you have to de-value a person during communication, you are motivated by fear instead of love.
- Remember that everyone you meet is a reflection of some part of you. If you feel rejected, you are rejecting yourself at some level, etc.
- Choose to leave toxic situations and toxic communication—know that anything less than nurturing and honor is abuse.

# CHAPTER SIX

## Letting Love In

## Principle #36

I am ready to give attention to what *I do want* in my relationship, rather than focus on what I do not want, as I remember that whatever I give my attention to grows.

As I am understanding myself more, knowing that my core issues have created my experiences… and as I am ready and willing to learn to speak and communicate in loving kindness, I also am ready to apply the laws of manifestation and attraction and I give myself permission to love deeply without fear.

This means that I am ready to give attention to what I do want to create in my relationship. How I am thinking and feeling has everything to do with what I am creating and experiencing. And, no matter why I am feeling like I am… or from which core issue my thoughts and feelings come from—I must make every effort I can to keep my focus on what I want in this relationship.

I will always get whatever I am thinking and *feeling* about, therefore, I choose to give energy to what I want in the form of feeling confident and secure that it will happen. If I am merely saying or writing about what I want, the universe hears me saying that I am not satisfied and that I am unhappy and therefore, more of the same thing keeps happening.

*So, when my relationship and communication challenges me—I must consciously become the Master of my feelings (after I express and release them)… do my best to BELIEVE AND FEEL good feelings about what is coming. As this may be a challenge, I must have a plan for how to do this, so I do not get caught giving a lot of attention to what I do not want. Because, when I am wishing or thinking that I want someone to change, I am actually reinforcing the experience, not allowing the new level of relationship to come into my life. Oh my gooness, I almost forgot this!*

# Principle #37

The key to experiencing freedom and real emotional intimacy is to love myself more and more deeply.

Learning about *Intimacy without Responsibility* really is a way of coming to understand that I am important, that I must have a voice, speak my truth, share my feelings, tell you what I need and honor myself. When I am a caretaker or someone wanting to save you or fix your life or circumstances, I am not loving myself so much. Because if I am focused on all of that, I do not have time for taking care of my own needs. My relationship with you, and you, and you… is completely about my relationship with me. *You* will always reflect my own feelings and treatment of myself.

That is why it is important to do the healing work on my core wounds, and to understand what a healthy relationship looks like. We must transform past programming and cellular imprints to increase our ability to choose. When we are holding old painful and negative core beliefs about ourselves and the world, our ability to choose diminishes.

*The key factor in all of this work is that I must learn to love myself deeply. Anyone and everyone in my life will match my love for myself. If someone is not loving me the way I think they should, then I, too am the one not loving me as I should. If someone is not treating me as a sacred being, then I am the one who is also not treating myself as a sacred being. It is as simple as that.*

*Today, I choose to do everything I can to love myself more deeply. I choose to do everything I can to treat myself as a sacred being… to continue to be conscious of my own feelings about myself, so that I can heal and transform everything that makes me feel less than! I get it. As I learn how to love myself deeply, I allow real, true, honest and sacred love in my life.*

## Principle #38

I commit to learning new ways to process what is happening in my world, so that I can love myself more and more.

*When I love myself deeply, I take good care of my inner Self. What does this mean? To love my inner self deeply means that I must observe my innermost thoughts, feelings and reactions to the behaviors of others, the world and myself.*

*Here are the steps I will take:*

1. Observe my thoughts and feelings as a conscious creator…
2. Feel my feelings…
3. Express my feelings…
4. Ask myself: What part of me am I rejecting or not loving… what part of me is holding shame or negative emotion about myself…how am I judging myself?
5. Become the Master of my emotions by finding a new thought that helps me feel better about the situation if my feeling and thoughts are of a painful or negative vibration…
6. Love myself and forgive myself (and others) for anything I wish I had not created, moving toward wholeness and joy as soon as I possibly can…
7. Be patient with myself each time, knowing this is a process…
8. Let go of judgment and remember that I am the creator…
9. Consciously practice loving myself…
10. I continue to realize that it is *all about me*. The world is matching *me*, and I am matching my experiences!

*I forgive myself this minute for any pain I have created for myself. I know that all is well, and I choose now to move to a feeling of love, knowing that I have really done the best that I could (and so have you). I will rise above my pain (after I express it) and remember that something good is coming!*

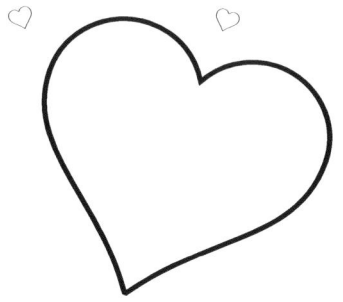

### Principle #39

How I process what is going on will give me the powerful ability to experience *freedom*.

*How I process whatever is going on is more important than what is going on. How I think and feel about what is happening with me and for me, is more important than the content of what is happening.*

*These are the beliefs that help me move toward higher consciousness in the midst of chaos and drama:*

1. Whatever is going on is part of my life drama and creation at some level—there to take me deeper to my true divine self.
2. Every problem is something I have brought into my energy field to help my soul evolve.
3. I am here on the earth to evolve my soul.
4. Every person and relationship in my life is here to teach me something important and help move me toward wholeness.
5. I am confident, secure and excited that all good things, people, places, experiences and successes are coming toward me now.
6. I can be the Master of my emotions right now!
7. All is well. Everything is okay.

*As I transform my painful and negative thoughts and feelings into power, hope, love, confidence and joy, I change my life… no matter if you do or not. That is* Intimacy without Responsibility, *and I love it!*

*I love to process whatever is going on with me in this way. I commit now to take the time to remember this way to think and feel about any kind of chaos, drama or trauma that is going on in my life. I am so grateful for this.*

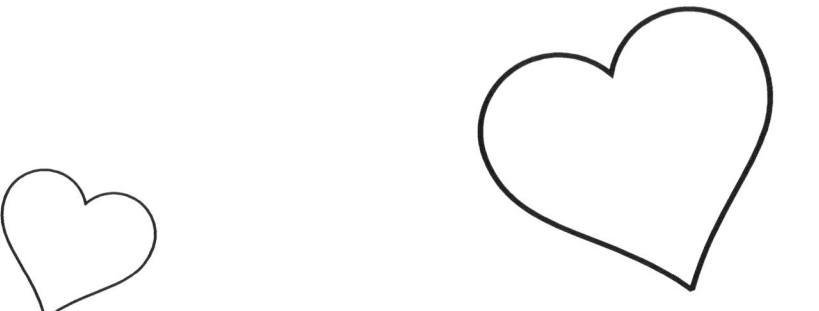

# Principle #40

I am ready and committed to *surrender* that which I have no control over. I am ready to let love in and experience a new kind of relationship with you, as I let go of *how* I can help or change you.

When I am helping you and thinking I know exactly how you must heal or be with me or others... I am the one who is manipulating and controlling. I have been in error, believing that I was doing this for your best interest.

I now know that all my best efforts for your healing and transformation has done nothing more than create a dependency on me—one in which you actually resent at some deep level.

I have thought I was doing the right thing, in the name of love! Really, I was acting out of my own fear. I was not letting love in, and allowing my own energy to diminish with the stress of wanting to control everything so you would be safe. Or really for me... that I would be safe.

If I am to love myself, and let love into my life in freeing, creative and heathy ways, I must let go of the effort to keep you or anyone else safe. I now know that when I do this, I stop you from connecting to the power of the universe and your own soul, to find your own path.

I have been contributing to your powerlessness all this time. Today, I am ready and committed to surrender this pattern. The time is right now for me to truly hand you over to the great power of your own soul and your own heart.

A part of me and my old brain, my old story, my own way of being with you... must die. I forgive myself for acting out of fear and old trauma in my own life. I surrender YOU now, that which I have never had control over.

## Principle #41

Everything I am experiencing is an illusion, therefore, I choose now to walk out of my old story, creating a new one complete with love, joy and peace.

I am the one who gives my life meaning... based on my learned beliefs and the way they are programmed in my brain, body/mind and spirit. Everyone else is doing the same thing. This is why we all have different reactions and thoughts and feelings to the same stimuli. How we were programmed from past pain and trauma, when we were born, where we were born, our past life experiences, womb, birth, soul memories and generations of patterns passing through the bloodline... create *me* in the now. And to complicate matters, there are several of *me!* I have several sub-personalities, and even they do not always get along.

So truly who is right or who is wrong? We are all living in our own real illusion, which we call our *reality*. Here are some other words for illusion:

> *a false idea or belief; something with a deceptive appearance or impression; a thing that is or is likely to be wrongly perceived or interpreted by the senses; delusion, misconception, false impression; fantasy, fancy, dream, self-deception; misperception, false appearance; mirage, hallucination, apparition, figment of the imagination...*

*Practicing* Intimacy without Responsibility *means that I honor the universal truth that reminds me—everything is really an illusion. At the end of the day, I am the actor in my personal movie and everyone else is part of the cast and crew. I choose now to write a new script, one that allows me to live in joy and peace. I also realize that you are the actor in your own reality and both of us really believe in our own! And, at times our realities do not match. That is okay. I will do my best to understand yours if you will do the same for me.*

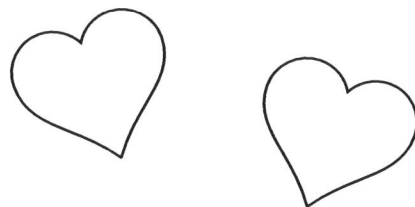

## Principle #42

As I consciously commit to confidence, security and an excitement about what kind of love, intimacy and relationship I can create now, and as I love myself more and more deeply, I experience a deep feeling of satisfaction, contentment, peace and joy.

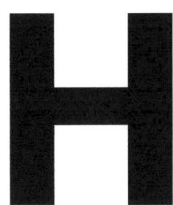ere are the tools required for experiencing *Intimacy without Responsibility*. They are the ways/practices that will transform old beliefs and habits…

1. Create a Conscious Intention based on new information about the joy of experiencing intimacy and deep love for another without responsibility for another person's happiness or success.
2. Write a new story. Really get clear about the kind of relationship you would like to experience. Allow yourself to believe that it can happen.
3. Intentionally surrender the old story and relationship patterns. Do the work you must do for healing and transforming your old story when needed.
4. Commit to a daily practice of imagining your new story, feeling what it will feel like… so to create new receptor sites in the brain for new behaviors, thoughts and feelings.
5. Be willing to change everything so you can really experience the joy of intimacy with another human being.
6. Become the Master of your emotions… consciously feeling, releasing, expressing and transforming insecurity, fear, anger and powerlessness to confidence, security and excitement about what love can really be.
7. Love yourself deeply so you will bring someone else toward you who will do the same thing.

*Yes, I commit now to a new story—my new storyline, and it is all about truly surrendering my old relationship pattern with you, and you, and maybe even you. I am ready for everything to change. I am ready to be the Master of my emotions and my life. I let go of fear and powerlessness. I am greatness!*

# CHAPTER SEVEN

## The Evolution of Love

## Principle #43

In this expanded, enlightened view, *Intimacy without Responsibility* is about love, freedom, trust and opening to the inner beloved—a me, you and we—that becomes a very sacred and powerful thing.

Relationship is the final healing ground… that place we have to test all that we have been working on in the personal growth process.

The evolution of love is that place where and when we are so in love with ourselves that we discover our *Inner Beloved*—our other half inside. Once we feel this, we can join with another person, without losing ourselves… and create a sacred enlightened relationship.

*Me* in an evolved and enlightened relationship is that piece of me that has lost the ego, that can be vulnerable and create from a powerful place of love, trust and power… the power to do what I might not be able to do alone—without fear of joining and letting go.

Intimacy without Responsibility *is about true love, real love—a divine love. It is truly patient and kind and open and trusting and synergistic and exciting without anger and ego and fear and anything that stops us from being who we are or anything that blocks us from our joy. Love evolved gives us the power to be and know and live in our greatness as me, and we!*

*So many times, I have done everything myself, and I notice how I want to lead and guide and direct and fix and even control. When I let go absolutely and become one with another soul in love, I actually have more freedom, more power, more uniqueness and a peace that is incredible. I am me. And I am you.*

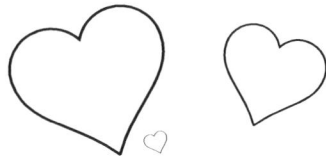

## Principle #44

*Intimacy without Responsibility* is an evolutionary process—transforming, unfolding, expanding and advancing my being.

The way we are in relationship becomes hardwired and we are neurochemically dependent on being with someone or having a situation be the *same*. We will always attract people who will act in certain ways to produce a chemical response in our bodies that we are familiar with. We live in a prison of our own past memories and habits. We become our state of mind and stay that way and therefore limit the possibilities for a new life, until and unless we do an intervention on our own minds and thoughts!

Albert Einstein said, *"You cannot solve a problem from the same mind that created it."* Brain research proves that this is absolutely true. We are all chemically addicted to the way we think! Whenever we repeat a thought, feeling or behavior, we create a complete neural network pattern, complete with its own receptor site that once imprinted, will beg/crave for more of that behavior.

*I do not want to keep doing the same old thing or having the same old result, which is exactly what happens when I close my mind and choose to think the same thoughts I chose yesterday. If I am having the same type experiences every day, it is because I am thinking the same thoughts from the same mind that thought the thoughts yesterday, and the day before, and the day before… and on and on.*

*I am choosing not to live my life in mediocrity—average, uninspired, indifferent, unexciting, unremarkable or run-of-the-mill. And, I certainly do not want this in my relationships. How exciting it will be to create a new mind!*

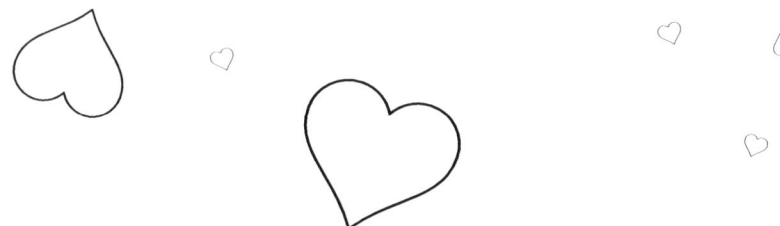

## Principle #45

I am engaging the evolution of love and enlightenment, as I open and change my mind.

**enlightenment** · noun *(Wikepedia)*
the action of enlightening or the state of being enlightened:

- the action or state of attaining or having attained spiritual knowledge or insight, in particular (in Buddhism) that awareness which frees a person from the cycle of rebirth; insight, understanding, awareness, wisdom, education, learning, knowledge; illumination, awakening, instruction, teaching; sophistication, advancement, development, open-mindedness, broad-mindedness; culture, refinement, cultivation, civilization.

*Yes! I continue to learn that my old mind will create the same old thing. I need to say that again and again. The key then, is not to change someone else but to change my own mind! When I change my mind, and hopefully create a new mind—I will have new neural networks that crave new experiences, dismantling the literal craving in my body for the old pattern— the old way of being in relationship with my beloved, my children, my parents, my colleagues and the earth.*

*Oh, how I crave to be in integrity with my world. The thing is, my mind is not always in integrity with my body… my actions do not always follow my intention, because my mind/body/brain is chemically connected to a different pattern.*

*I am committed to enlightenment and to practice what I learn! Practice, practice, practice, practice, practice... and on and on... until I have a new mind. The only thing I really have to change is everything!*

## Principle #46

If I am ever truly to experience enlightened relationship, I must be willing to practice some kind of mind intervention...
a way of changing my mind and creating a new one.

The *Intimacy without Responsibility Mind Intervention Practices* consist of creating first an enlightened, deep, loving relationship in your mind. Write about it. Become aware of how this relationship is different or similar to past experiences with your love partner. Those aspects of the relationship you desire that are *not* part of your past experience will be the part needing chemical re-programming in your body/mind. Get very clear about this.

Next, create a written scenario that describes your loving relationship. Talk about new ways of thinking, feeling and being… and this is as much about *you* as your partner. Remember, you are the one that is re-programming. Your partner will change, when you change. Or, you will attract that person or relationship once you have a place for it in your biochemistry.

Know that if your partner goes to great lengths to change and *you* have *not changed* your thinking, feeling and being—eventually you will experience the old pattern because that is all you can experience!

Lastly, commit to imagining this scenario *every day* for seven weeks at least one hour day in meditation. This practice will change your life!

*Whenever I am thinking the same limited thoughts, I am continuing the same old habits and ways of being. If I am to advance and move to a higher level of being, I must welcome new thoughts, ideas and experiences—think outside my same old box. I commit to the evolution of love.*

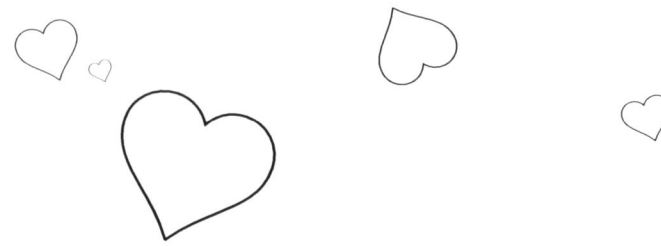

## Principle #47

People who approach love and relationship from higher perspectives and higher mind are moving toward the evolution of love and will experience enlightened relationship.

*I choose now to understand my relationships in a more evolved, advanced manner. I choose to open my mind to new possibilities and ways of thinking and being. The following thoughts are part of my mind intervention practice. I choose to believe:*

- That I am the creator of my experiences…
- That I have everything to do with the joy and pain in my life…
- That everything around me is a mirror of my unconscious thoughts, feelings, ways of doing and being stored in my mind/body…
- That I can be the master of my thoughts and feelings…
- That what I am experiencing right now is a familiar pattern – one that is neuro-chemically imprinted in my brain/body/mind …
- That my perceptions come from my past memories and experiences …
- That I am emotionally addicted to these perceptions because my brain chemistry craves the same experience…
- That I am willing to discover the unconscious habits that are now stored in my mind/body…
- That I am ready to do whatever it takes to do my own mind intervention and create a new reality…
- That I am ready to evolve my being, my brain, my life and my relationships…
- That I am ready to create and activate new neural networks so I can think, feel, act and become all that I choose to be…
- That I am ready to experience a completely new level of love and enlightened relationship…
- That I can apply these principles to everything in my life…

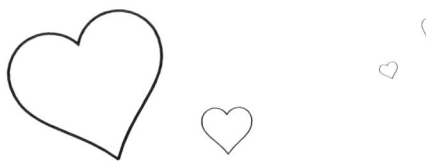

## Principle #48

Enlightened relationship and the ability to practice *Intimacy without Responsibility* is about commitment to my soul's evolution.

Enlightened relationship is about commitment to a process that sits deep within my soul—one in which I become willing to really change my perception of things, maybe even everything.

In just the perfect moment, this information will present itself to the one who is ready. Until then, one can do nothing else but think the same old thing and live in the same old "reality". I suppose there is that right moment for everyone… that time when we really get something at a new level of consciousness. Not everyone is ready for the evolution of love or *Intimacy without Responsibility*.

Evolution is not about accepting mediocrity or abuse. Higher consciousness is not about condoning unhealthy or dysfunctional behavior in our loved ones that hurt us. Evolution and higher consciousness is about *how we process* what happens… how we communicate our feelings, and how we take responsibility to see our part in all the experiences of our life.

*Well, I finally get it! The brain chemistry studies and written works really opened my mind to understanding why I have been unable to follow through with healthy actions, communication and higher ways of being with all my love and close relationships. I thank the Universe for this.*

Intimacy without Responsibility *is an evolutionary process, helping us know ourselves more deeply and honoring the great mystery of all that is. I continue to commit myself always to learning more and perceiving all my relationships, even those that have hurt deeply—as sacred.*

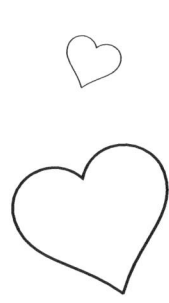

## Principle #49

Every part of all my relationships are forever changed, as I practice *Intimacy without Responsibility* and remember that *all is well*.

*Intimacy Without Responsibility* has been a study about learning to be in relationship without taking responsibility for another person's feelings or pain or even their success or joy! *Freedom in relationship is about becoming very clear about my own codependency—the roles I continue to play with others... my intimate partner, as well as family, friends and colleagues.*

*Intimacy without Responsibility* has been about practicing the art and skill of freedom in relationship... moving toward more love and *care for self*. *I realize that when I truly heal and take care of ALL of my own issues, I are able to love more deeply.*

*Intimacy without Responsibility* has also been about the mystery and sacred space that relationship takes us. This work honors the universal truth that tells us: *Every relationship I have is mirroring something about me that is wanting to come up into consciousness for my healing and transformation... for my wholeness and the evolution of my soul. And whenever I have a problem or issue with you, I have an opportunity to heal and transform something inside me... like an unresolved old wound or trauma, something I lost, something I always needed, or something I do not even know—that has all been imprinted neurochemically in my mind/body.*

*Now I know that every person I attract in my life is a part of my wholeness, a missing piece of the healing puzzle—that no matter what happens in this relationship, I am healing more because I am choosing to view every part of this relationship as a sacred thing moving me toward higher consciousness, the evolution of love and the evolution of my being.*

# EPILOGUE

And

*Today I am committed to emotional intimacy with others—with you... which means that I will speak my truth, be real, feel my feelings, share my feelings, not hold back how I am feeling about you or me or the world AND commit to my personal mission and purpose. I will give myself permission to discover who I am AND what my personal path is if I do not know yet.*

*I give myself permission this day to let go of any toxic relationship and all toxic communication in my life. I choose to live and walk a path of peace. I choose to communicate in loving kindness, aware that my perceptions come from my belief system... AND that your perceptions come from yours, and we may not agree. That is okay with me, as long as we can communicate in a way that honors us both.*

*I give myself permission this day to stop taking care of you or trying to protect you or trying to keep you alive. AND I finally realize that you may not want what I want for you, that you have the right to choose your own path completely, AND I am ready to surrender the illusion of control I thought I had.*

*I commit this day to doing healing work on my own core wounds so that I do not project them on you or blame you for whatever is going on. AND I know now that you are a mirror of my core wounds and issues, things I lost, my fears, my shame, and parts of my soul.*

*Today, I shall honor your right to do your life the way you choose... to be who you are, to let you be who you are in all ways. AND, I have the right and the freedom to decide if I shall join you or not as I practice loving and taking care of my Self more and more, from this day evermore.*

*I ask myself this day to face my fears and rejoice, to look my fears straight in the eye and do whatever it is I need to do for myself to create safe boundaries for me, even if that means letting go or cutting cords of enmeshment with you. No matter what, I thank you for mirroring all my core issues for me. If I must, I let you go in love and I commit to my own new mind.*

*AND, I give myself permission this day to let love in my life in ways I have not yet experienced. I commit to honor my own body, mind and spirit. I shall put myself first, knowing that this will enhance my love for you, because I will have great energy to love you better when I take care of myself. I know now that I cannot love you if I do not love myself.*

*I give myself permission this day to be a powerful human being, moving forward on my own soul's journey toward wholeness, knowing that all my experiences and relationships have been my teachers—painful and joyful AND that everything has happened for a powerful purpose. I am ready to experience enlightened relationship AND the evolution of love.*

*AND I commit to practicing* Intimacy without Responsibility. *I will continue to discover how my feelings and thoughts create my reality and will adjust my mind program as needed. I have the evolution technology now, and I commit to continued practice, practice, practice.*

*It is my wish that you will join me on this relationship journey. Together, with our higher vibrational selves, we can help change the world and teach this kind of peace to all.*

*AND so it is!*

About the Author

*I am here to help you become
all you are meant to be.*

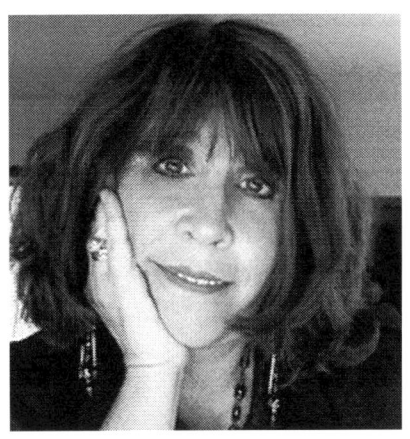

**W**endyne Limber, MA, LMFT, RDT/BCT is the founder of Solutions Center for Personal Growth and Soul Studies Institute in Stuart, FL. She is a Florida Licensed Marriage and Family Therapist, Registered Drama Therapist and Board Certified Trainer of Drama Therapists.

In 1990, Wendyne created *The Imagination Process,*™ a 21-week healing and transformational program integrating old and new psychology, Eastern and Western thought, spiritual and human truths with drama therapy and the Arts for a healing journey into the mystery of psyche and the universe. *The Imagination Process*™ has continued to evolve over the last 20 years, helping many people heal old wounds, habits and behavior patterns, express and release feelings and trauma, face fear, integrate shadow, learn a language of power, and become the architect of their life design! Wendyne created *Intimacy Without Responsibility* as a book, a workshop, a process and way of being in relationship with others.

**T**hank you for reading and working with my book, Intimacy Without Responsibility, *a book in which I present to you writings and universal principles illuminating the secrets of real love and intimacy. This book was inspired by couples who were fearful of emotional connection, even terrified that they would be eaten up by the other, obligated and responsible for the happiness of their loved ones. Or in some cases, a person felt completely the opposite—abandoned, dependent and petrified of being alone, feeling needy and wanting to be wanted, touched and appreciated.*

*I am happy to report that upon engaging the healing process of* Intimacy Without Responsibility, *couples such as these came to the middle... allowed themselves to fall in love with Self and then each other again, learning that, indeed, they are responsible only for their own soul's evolutionary journey, and that one can consciously move toward wholeness and the evolution of love in a way that brings joy and peace in all relationships.*

*As I began writing and teaching these principles, I activated my own intense personal healing journey... all about codependency with my children and grand-children. Oh, how I have had to be the living teaching! Writing and living this book feels like a completion for me... as I surrender old relationship patterns that no longer serve me or anyone else.*

...

Please visit the website link for *Intimacy Without Responsibility* if you are interested in purchasing this book for you or someone else, discovering other seminar dates or for general information. Also included are website links for anyone interested in participating in one of Wendyne Limber's healing programs, groups, or educational offerings.

**Solutions Center for Personal Growth** • www.solutionsforhealing.com
*A healing center in Stuart, Florida, where we are guiding and loving people to their highest*

*potential and being.*

**The Imagination Process™** • www.theimaginationprogram.com
*A 21-week healing program for healing and transformation.*

**Imagine Drama Therapy™** • www.imaginedramatherapy.com
*A traning program for anyone interested in becoming a Registered Drama Therapist.*

**Soul Studies Institute** • www.soulstudies.com
*Our 501 (c)3 not-for-profit school, freeing the creative spirit with transpersonal education and the creative arts; continuing education for mental health professionals.*

**More About Wendyne Limber** • www.wendynelimber.com

# ACKNOWLEDGEMENTS

I thank all the incredible, beautiful people I work with, who believe in me and have always honored the healing work I so love.

Thank you, Charlie, for pushing me to write this book. There was just something about how you talked to me that night, as we all sat overlooking the ocean—sharing, planning and envisioning our future. I will never forget your words... and the inspiration they provided me all this time. This is that first real book.

Thank you, Petrina, for being my incredibly talented and unique sister and editor of this work. Thanks for always believing in me. You have taught me so much about writing, words and family relovingships (you even said I could make up a new word)! I am glad you are a master of the English language, a gifted writer, therapist, actor and human woman.

Thank you, Pamela Heartsong, for trusting me from the very beginning of our relovingship and for always being there for me, giving and walking with me through the middle of the many aspects of my life and work. You are the wind beneath my wings so many times.

Thank you, Kathy and John, for having an issue that needed the creation of this book and work, *Intimacy Without Responsibility*. Our time together working these principles was truly a spiritual experience for me, and I was the honored guest at your healing. Thank you, Ted, for being so fearful of intimacy that I had to figure out a way to help you open your heart and trust that love is not about taking responsibility for some helpless woman. You proved that the work can change anyone! And thank you, Holly, for working on your Self, when you and Ted were not doing the work together. We truly learn that we do not do the process, rather the process does us.

I thank all those who have participated in the *Intimacy Without Responsibility* (Advanced

Possibilities Training) class. You have always inspired me to be the therapist that I am, and I mean it when I say… You complete me (not a principle from the book)! How incredible it is for me to sit and teach and laugh and cry sacred tears with you all this time.

And thanks to all you artists and graphic designers who helped me make the book feel good. Thanks, Sam, for the heart, and Maryanne for the great looking postcard, and Aaron for staying up half the night at the last minute creating all the book design and other various products.

Thanks to everyone on the Soul Studies Institute Board of Directors who assisted me with this project and the first *Intimacy Without Responsibility Adventure Seminar*, especially Barb, who coached me on every step I needed to accomplish my goals; and to Michelle for taking responsibility for getting out the word about our work; and to Erin for your genius, knowledge and ideas; and Kathy for your everlasting love and support.

Lastly, I thank my children and grandchildren for most likely agreeing to come to the earth as my children, to help me evolve my soul through all the joy and pain we have experienced together. This book has been my journey through co-dependency. I know I have birthed a new me because of it, and this will help others do the same. Thank you for your part. I love you all so deeply. Thank you my husband, Jim, for being you. We have always lived a life of intimacy without responsibility, and that is why I love you so much. And you will have to read this book to find out what I am talking about!

And so it is that I am not alone any more. I hope all of you will love this work as much as I do, and that it will move you toward deep emotional intimacy and the evolution of love in your life.

Printed in Poland
by Amazon Fulfillment
Poland Sp. z o.o., Wrocław